# HORMONAL BALANCE DIET FOR WOMEN

A Holistic Journey to Reclaim Vitality, Sex Drive, Lose Weight, Health, and Hormonal Harmony With Delicious Recipes and Meal Plan

Dr. Wendy Fuhrman S.

# ABOUT THE AUTHOR:

Dr. Wendy Fuhrman S. is a prominent figure in the field of women's health and nutrition. Her life's work has been dedicated to empowering women to take charge of their well-being, focusing on the transformative potential of proper nutrition.

Dr. Wendy Fuhrman S. has earned recognition as a trailblazer in women's health. Her unwavering dedication to improving the lives of women has made her a leading figure in the field. Over the years, she has served as a strong advocate for women's health, offering guidance, expertise, and unwavering support to women from all walks of life.

With a degree in Nutrition and Dietetics, Dr. Wendy Fuhrman S. possesses the knowledge and skills necessary to guide women on their path to optimal health. Her profound understanding of the intricate relationship between nutrition and hormonal balance has allowed her to create life-changing strategies that have positively impacted countless women.

Dr. Wendy Fuhrman S.'s core mission is to help women achieve hormonal balance and regain their vitality. Her holistic approach to health underscores the importance of nurturing the body, mind, and spirit. Through her work, she has empowered women to overcome challenges such as PCOS, endometriosis, menopause, and more, all while promoting a sense of well-being and equilibrium.

As a respected author, Dr. Wendy Fuhrman S. has authored several influential books, including the best-selling "Hormonal Balance Diet for Women." Her writings serve as guiding beacons, equipping women with the knowledge and practical tools necessary to lead healthier, more fulfilling lives.

With her guidance, you can embark on a journey toward renewed vitality, balanced hormones, and overall well-being. Place your trust in her expertise, draw inspiration from her passion, and allow her to be your partner in achieving a healthier and happier life.

# TABLE OF CONTENTS

# INTRODUCTION

Welcome to a transformative journey that marries the ancient wisdom of nutrition with the latest in hormonal health research. As a leading expert in women's health and hormonal balance, I've witnessed firsthand the profound impact that diet can have on our well-being. The key to unlocking this potential lies not just in what we eat, but in understanding the intricate dance of hormones that governs our bodies. To illuminate this path, allow me to share the story of Miss Augusta, a case study that epitomizes the struggles and triumphs many women face on the road to hormonal harmony.

Miss Augusta, a vibrant teacher in her early thirties, came to me burdened by symptoms that many would dismiss as the tolls of a busy life: fatigue that no amount of sleep could erase, unpredictable moods that felt like emotional rollercoasters, and a metabolism that seemed to have ground to a halt. Like so many, she had been told that these were simply the cards she'd been dealt, a notion she bravely challenged in pursuit of a better quality of life.

Our journey began with a deep dive into her lifestyle, from the foods that filled her plate to the rhythms of her daily life. It became clear that Miss Augusta's diet, though rich in variety, was inadvertently throwing her hormonal balance into disarray. Her story, while unique, is not uncommon. It echoes the experiences of countless women who navigate through life's stages, from the tumultuous teenage years to the transformative phases of menopause, often without realizing the power they hold over their hormonal health.

This book is dedicated to every woman who, like Miss Augusta, seeks not just to survive but to thrive. Through her story, we'll explore how the principles of the Hormonal Balance Diet can serve as a beacon of hope and a roadmap to reclaiming your health. You'll discover the profound connection between what you eat and how you feel, think, and live. This is not just a diet; it's a revolution in how we approach women's health, offering a holistic strategy that goes beyond mere symptom management to address the root causes of hormonal imbalance.

Miss Augusta's journey from confusion to clarity, from frustration to empowerment, is a testament to the resilience of the human spirit and the healing power of food. As we turn the pages, remember that her story could be anyone's. Whether you're grappling with specific health challenges or simply seeking to optimize your well-being, the insights and strategies you'll find here are your allies.

As we embark on this journey together, I invite you to keep an open mind and a hopeful heart. The path to hormonal balance is as much about nourishment as it is about discovery—of the foods that fuel you, the practices that ground you, and the lifestyle changes that transform you. Welcome to the Hormonal Balance Diet for Women, where your journey to wellness begins.

# CHAPTER 1

## UNDERSTANDING YOUR HORMONES

### The Role of Hormones in Women's Health

Hormones are the silent orchestrators of your body's functions. In women, these chemical messengers play a pivotal role in maintaining overall health and well-being. Imagine them as the conductors of an intricate symphony, ensuring that every instrument (organ) in your body plays in harmony.

Hormones are secreted by various glands throughout the body, including the pituitary, thyroid, adrenal, and ovaries. They regulate a wide array of functions, such as metabolism, mood, reproduction, and even the immune system. But what's particularly fascinating is their role in women's health.

For women, hormones govern everything from the menstrual cycle to pregnancy and menopause. They influence your energy levels, skin condition, and emotional state. Estrogen, progesterone, and testosterone are among the major players in this hormonal symphony.

Estrogen, often dubbed the "female hormone," is responsible for the development of secondary sexual characteristics, like breast development and a widening of the hips during puberty. It also regulates the menstrual cycle and plays a role in bone health.

Progesterone complements estrogen, ensuring the menstrual cycle proceeds smoothly and preparing the uterus for pregnancy. It's the hormone that rises during the second half of the menstrual cycle and declines if pregnancy doesn't occur, triggering menstruation.

Testosterone isn't exclusive to men. Women have it too, albeit in smaller amounts. It's essential for muscle strength, bone density, and libido. When imbalanced, it can lead to changes in mood and energy levels.

Understanding these hormonal roles is crucial because imbalances can result in a range of health issues. Hormonal disorders, such as polycystic ovary syndrome (PCOS) and endometriosis, are common among women and can lead to fertility problems, irregular periods, and discomfort. By comprehending the delicate hormonal dance within your body, you're better equipped to recognize when something is amiss and seek appropriate care.

## Key Hormones and Their Functions

Now, let's delve deeper into the major hormones at play in women's health and their functions.

Estrogen: As mentioned earlier, estrogen is responsible for the development of female secondary sexual characteristics. It thickens the uterine lining during the menstrual cycle and declines before menstruation begins. During pregnancy, estrogen levels surge, supporting fetal development. In menopause, declining estrogen can lead to symptoms like hot flashes and mood swings.

Progesterone: Progesterone's primary role is to prepare the uterus for pregnancy. It maintains the uterine lining during the second half of the menstrual cycle. If fertilization doesn't occur, progesterone levels drop, triggering menstruation. It also helps maintain pregnancy and prevents uterine contractions during gestation.

Testosterone: Often associated with men, testosterone is essential for women too. It supports muscle and bone health, regulates libido, and plays a role in mood and cognitive function. While women have lower testosterone levels than men, it's still a critical hormone for overall well-being.

Thyroid Hormones (T3 and T4): These hormones, produced by the thyroid gland, control metabolism. They influence energy levels, body temperature, and weight. An imbalance in thyroid hormones can lead to fatigue, weight fluctuations, and mood changes.

Cortisol: Produced by the adrenal glands, cortisol is the "stress hormone." It helps the body respond to stress by increasing glucose levels in the bloodstream. Chronic stress can lead to cortisol imbalances, affecting sleep, mood, and immune function.

Understanding these key hormones and their functions provides a foundation for recognizing when they're not working as they should. Hormonal imbalances can manifest in various ways, from irregular periods and mood swings to fertility issues and fatigue.

## Signs of Hormonal Imbalance

Hormonal imbalances can disrupt the delicate equilibrium of your body, leading to a range of symptoms. Recognizing these signs is crucial for early intervention and achieving hormonal balance.

1. Irregular Menstrual Cycles: One of the most common signs of hormonal imbalance in women is irregular periods. This can manifest as missed periods, heavy bleeding, or unusually long cycles.

2. Mood Swings and Emotional Changes: Hormones have a profound impact on mood. Fluctuations can lead to mood swings, irritability, anxiety, or even depression.

3. Unexplained Weight Changes: Hormonal imbalances, particularly in thyroid hormones, can lead to unexplained weight gain or loss.

4. Acne and Skin Changes: Hormones influence skin health. Imbalances can lead to acne outbreaks or changes in skin texture and tone.

5. Fatigue and Low Energy: Hormonal disruptions often result in persistent fatigue, even with adequate rest.

6. Changes in Libido: Shifts in testosterone levels can affect sexual desire and satisfaction.

7. Hair and Nail Changes: Hormonal imbalances may cause hair thinning or changes in nail health.

8. Sleep Disturbances: Cortisol imbalances can disrupt sleep patterns, leading to insomnia or poor sleep quality.

9. Fertility Issues: Hormonal disorders like PCOS can lead to fertility problems and difficulty conceiving.

10. Hot Flashes and Night Sweats: During menopause, declining estrogen levels can trigger hot flashes and night sweats.

Recognizing these signs is the first step toward addressing hormonal imbalances. It's essential to consult a healthcare professional for proper diagnosis and treatment tailored to your specific needs.

# CHAPTER 2

## THE CONNECTION BETWEEN DIET AND HORMONES

### How Food Affects Your Hormones

The relationship between food and hormones is a complex and fascinating one. Our bodies rely on a delicate balance of hormones to regulate various physiological processes, from metabolism to mood. What many don't realize is that the foods we consume can have a significant impact on these hormonal systems.

Let's begin by understanding the role of insulin, a hormone produced by the pancreas. When we consume carbohydrates, especially those with a high glycemic index, our blood sugar levels spike. In response, the pancreas releases insulin to help cells absorb the excess sugar. This is a normal process, but when it occurs frequently due to a diet high in refined carbs and sugars, it can lead to insulin resistance. This condition, closely associated with obesity and type 2 diabetes, disrupts the hormonal balance and can have long-term health consequences.

Similarly, dietary fats play a crucial role in hormone production. Healthy fats, such as those found in avocados, nuts, and fatty fish, are essential for synthesizing hormones. On the other hand, a diet high in trans fats and saturated fats can lead to inflammation and interfere with hormone production.

Another critical aspect is protein intake. Amino acids, the building blocks of proteins, are necessary for the synthesis of hormones like insulin and growth hormone. A diet lacking in adequate protein can lead to hormonal imbalances, affecting muscle growth, immune function, and more.

Furthermore, micronutrients such as vitamins and minerals are essential for hormone regulation. For instance, vitamin D is known to influence the production of sex hormones, and deficiencies can lead to hormonal issues. Zinc, another micronutrient, plays a role in the production of thyroid hormones, crucial for metabolism and overall well-being.

## Nutrients Essential for Hormonal Balance

Hormonal balance hinges on the availability of specific nutrients that act as building blocks and regulators for various hormones. Let's explore some of these essential nutrients and their roles in maintaining hormonal equilibrium.

- Omega-3 Fatty Acids: These healthy fats, abundant in fatty fish like salmon and walnuts, play a crucial role in regulating inflammation and supporting hormone production. Omega-

3s are associated with improved insulin sensitivity, which is vital for overall hormonal balance.

- Vitamin D: Often referred to as the "sunshine vitamin," vitamin D is critical for hormone health. It influences the production of sex hormones like estrogen and testosterone. Adequate sun exposure and dietary sources like fatty fish and fortified foods can help maintain optimal vitamin D levels.

- Fiber: Dietary fiber, found in fruits, vegetables, and whole grains, can aid in hormonal balance by promoting steady blood sugar levels. High-fiber diets are linked to reduced insulin resistance and a lower risk of type 2 diabetes.

- Magnesium: This mineral is involved in over 300 enzymatic reactions in the body, including those related to hormone synthesis and regulation. Nuts, seeds, and leafy greens are excellent sources of magnesium.

- B Vitamins: The B-vitamin complex, including B6 and B12, plays a role in neurotransmitter synthesis and can impact mood-regulating hormones like serotonin. Incorporating lean meats, fish, and leafy greens into your diet can ensure an adequate intake of B vitamins.

- Antioxidants: Vitamins C and E, along with selenium, are antioxidants that protect cells from oxidative stress. This protection extends to hormone-producing glands, helping to maintain their function. Citrus fruits, nuts, and seeds are rich in these antioxidants.

- Iodine: Iodine is essential for the production of thyroid hormones, which regulate metabolism. Seafood and iodized salt are common sources of iodine.

- Iron: Iron is critical for the production of hemoglobin, which carries oxygen in the blood. Hormones like erythropoietin are involved in regulating iron levels in the body.

Understanding the importance of these nutrients in hormonal balance underscores the significance of a well-rounded diet. By including a variety of nutrient-dense foods in your meals, you can ensure your body has the raw materials it needs to maintain optimal hormone function.

## Foods to Embrace and Avoid

Now that we've explored how food affects hormones and the essential nutrients for hormonal balance, let's delve into the specific foods to include in your diet and those to limit or avoid.

**Colorful Vegetables:**

- Leafy Greens: Vegetables like spinach, kale, and Swiss chard are rich in vitamins, minerals, and antioxidants. They provide essential nutrients such as vitamin K, which plays a role in hormone regulation, and magnesium, which supports insulin sensitivity.

- Cruciferous Vegetables: Broccoli, cauliflower, Brussels sprouts, and cabbage are members of the cruciferous family. They contain compounds called indole-3-carbinol and sulforaphane, which aid in the detoxification of estrogen, a crucial aspect of hormonal balance.

**Lean Proteins:**

- Poultry: Skinless chicken and turkey breasts are excellent sources of lean protein. Protein is essential for the production of hormones and enzymes.

- Fatty Fish: Salmon, mackerel, and trout provide omega-3 fatty acids, which reduce inflammation and support hormonal health. Additionally, these fish are rich in vitamin D, essential for hormone regulation.

- Plant-Based Proteins: Tofu, tempeh, and legumes like lentils and chickpeas are plant-based protein sources that offer a combination of protein and fiber. They help stabilize blood sugar levels, reducing the risk of insulin spikes.

**Healthy Fats:**

- Avocado: Avocados are a prime source of monounsaturated fats, which have anti-inflammatory properties. They also contain vitamin E, important for hormonal balance.

- Olive Oil: Extra virgin olive oil is a staple of the Mediterranean diet and is associated with reduced inflammation and improved insulin sensitivity.

- Nuts and Seeds: Almonds, walnuts, flaxseeds, and chia seeds provide healthy fats and fiber. They are rich in antioxidants and support hormone synthesis.

**Whole Grains:**

- Quinoa: This whole grain is not only high in fiber but also a complete protein source. It helps regulate blood sugar levels and provides essential amino acids.

- Brown Rice: Unlike white rice, brown rice is a whole grain that retains its bran and germ layers, offering more fiber and nutrients. It promotes stable energy levels.

- Oats: Oats are a fantastic source of soluble fiber, which slows down the absorption of carbohydrates and helps maintain steady blood sugar levels.

**Fruits:**

- Berries: Blueberries, strawberries, and raspberries are packed with antioxidants known as polyphenols. They combat oxidative stress and support overall health.

- Citrus Fruits: Oranges, grapefruits, and lemons are high in vitamin C, which can enhance immune function and aid in the detoxification of hormones.

**Foods to Limit or Avoid:**

**Processed Sugars:**

- Sodas: Sugary soft drinks are loaded with refined sugars that cause rapid spikes in blood sugar levels. Over time, this can lead to insulin resistance and hormonal imbalance.

- Candies and Desserts: Foods high in refined sugars and artificial sweeteners should be consumed in moderation or avoided altogether. They contribute to sugar cravings and metabolic disruptions.

**Trans Fats:**

- Fast Food: Fried foods commonly found in fast-food chains often contain trans fats. These fats promote inflammation and interfere with hormone regulation.

- Packaged Snacks: Many packaged snacks like potato chips and microwave popcorn contain trans fats. Always check labels for partially hydrogenated oils, a common source of trans fats.

**Excessive Caffeine:**

- Coffee: While moderate coffee consumption can be part of a healthy diet, excessive caffeine intake may elevate cortisol levels, the body's primary stress hormone. Limit caffeine to a moderate level that suits your individual tolerance.

**Alcohol:**

- Excessive Alcohol: Chronic alcohol consumption can disrupt the balance of sex hormones, leading to irregular menstrual cycles and other hormonal issues. If you choose to consume alcohol, do so in moderation.

**Processed Foods:**

- Highly Processed Snacks: Chips, crackers, and pre-packaged snacks often contain additives and preservatives that may disrupt hormonal function. Opt for whole, minimally processed alternatives.

**Artificial Sweeteners:**

- Diet Sodas: While marketed as a low-calorie option, diet sodas contain artificial sweeteners like aspartame and saccharin, which may have unforeseen effects on hormones. Water or herbal tea are better beverage choices.

CHAPTER 3:

THE BASICS OF THE HORMONAL BALANCE DIET

Before we delve into the specifics of the Hormonal Balance Diet, it's crucial to understand the foundational principles that underpin this dietary approach. This chapter is designed to equip you with the essential knowledge needed to embark on your journey toward hormonal balance through nutrition.

In the modern world, hormonal imbalances have become increasingly prevalent among women of all ages. Factors such as stress, poor dietary choices, environmental toxins, and sedentary lifestyles can all disrupt the delicate hormonal symphony within our bodies. The Hormonal Balance Diet offers a holistic solution, rooted in science, to address these imbalances.

## Principles of the Hormonal Balance Diet

The Hormonal Balance Diet is founded on a set of principles that guide your food choices and meal planning. These principles are not just about what you eat but also about when and how you eat. Let's explore each principle in detail:

Whole Foods Emphasis: The cornerstone of the Hormonal Balance Diet is a focus on whole, unprocessed foods. These foods are rich in essential nutrients, fiber, and phytonutrients, all of which play crucial roles in hormonal health. We'll delve into the benefits of whole foods and provide practical tips on incorporating them into your diet.

Balanced Macronutrients: Achieving hormonal balance requires a careful balance of macronutrients—carbohydrates, proteins, and fats. You'll learn how each macronutrient influences your hormones and discover the ideal ratios to support your health goals. We'll also debunk common myths about fats and carbohydrates.

Glycemic Control: The Hormonal Balance Diet places a strong emphasis on controlling the glycemic index of your meals. You'll understand why stabilizing blood sugar levels is pivotal for hormonal health, and we'll provide strategies to achieve this through your dietary choices.

Nutrient Timing: When you eat can be just as important as what you eat. We'll explore the concept of nutrient timing, including the benefits of intermittent fasting and meal timing for hormonal balance. You'll gain insights into how to synchronize your meals with your body's natural rhythms.

Mindful Eating: Mindfulness is a key component of the Hormonal Balance Diet. We'll delve into the importance of mindful eating practices, including listening to your body's hunger and fullness cues, reducing stress during meals, and savoring each bite.

Hydration: Proper hydration is often underestimated in its impact on hormonal health. You'll discover why staying adequately hydrated is essential and how to make hydration a part of your daily routine.

## How to Personalize Your Hormonal Balance Diet

Personalization is at the heart of the Hormonal Balance Diet. Recognizing that every woman is unique, with individual hormonal profiles and health objectives, is fundamental to achieving optimal results. In this section, we will explore the art of tailoring the Hormonal Balance Diet to your specific needs and goals.

### Assessing Your Hormonal Health

Before embarking on any dietary plan, it's crucial to gain insights into your current hormonal status. This knowledge will serve as the foundation upon which you can build your personalized Hormonal Balance Diet. Here's how to assess your hormonal health:

Self-Assessment Tools: We'll provide you with a range of self-assessment tools that allow you to gauge your hormonal well-being. These tools encompass various aspects of your health, from your menstrual cycle and mood to energy levels and sleep quality. By tracking and analyzing your responses, you'll start to paint a clearer picture of your hormonal landscape.

Hormone Testing: For a more precise evaluation, consider hormone testing. Blood tests, saliva tests, or urine tests can provide detailed information about your hormone levels. Consulting with a healthcare professional is advisable for interpreting these results accurately. We'll guide you on how to initiate these tests and what to expect from them.

Consulting a Healthcare Professional: If you have existing hormonal imbalances or health concerns, consulting a healthcare professional, such as an endocrinologist or a naturopathic doctor, can be invaluable. They can perform specialized tests and provide expert guidance tailored to your unique circumstances.

Once you've gathered information about your hormonal health, you'll have a clearer understanding of where your imbalances lie. This knowledge is the first step toward personalizing your Hormonal Balance Diet.

**Customizing Your Nutrient Ratios**

With insights into your hormonal health, you can begin to customize the macronutrient ratios of your diet. The Hormonal Balance Diet recognizes that there is no one-size-fits-all approach to nutrition. Depending on your specific hormonal imbalances or goals, such as weight management, fertility, or managing PCOS (Polycystic Ovary Syndrome), you can adjust your diet accordingly:

Balancing Carbohydrates: Carbohydrates play a significant role in hormonal balance. Depending on your needs, you can adjust the types and amounts of carbohydrates you consume. For example, if you're struggling with insulin resistance, a lower-carb approach may be beneficial. We'll provide you with guidance on choosing the right carbohydrates for your goals.

Protein for Hormonal Health: Protein is essential for hormone production and repair. The Hormonal Balance Diet offers recommendations on protein sources and quantities to support your specific hormonal requirements. Whether you're aiming for muscle maintenance, weight loss, or improved energy, we'll help you personalize your protein intake.

Fats and Hormones: Dietary fats are integral to hormonal health. Different fats have distinct effects on hormones. We'll demystify the role of fats in your diet, helping you choose the right fats for hormonal balance and overall well-being.

Micro and Macronutrient Ratios: Beyond individual macronutrients, we'll guide you in optimizing the overall ratio of carbohydrates, proteins, and fats in your daily meals. Achieving the right balance is key to hormonal harmony.

## Adapting for Life Phases

Hormonal needs evolve throughout a woman's life, from the tumultuous years of puberty to the transformative stages of pregnancy and menopause. The Hormonal Balance Diet recognizes the importance of adapting your dietary approach to these different life phases:

Puberty and Adolescence: Young women experiencing puberty may face hormonal fluctuations. The Hormonal Balance Diet can provide support during this transitional phase, helping to manage symptoms and establish a foundation for lifelong hormonal health.

Fertility and Pregnancy: For women aiming to conceive or currently pregnant, nutritional needs change significantly. We'll discuss how to adapt your diet to optimize fertility and ensure a healthy pregnancy.

Menopause and Beyond: Menopause brings its unique hormonal challenges. The Hormonal Balance Diet offers strategies for managing menopausal symptoms and promoting overall well-being during this life phase.

Post-Menopause: Beyond menopause, hormonal health remains a priority. We'll explore how to sustain hormonal balance as you age gracefully.

## Food Sensitivities and Allergies

Many women have food sensitivities or allergies that can exacerbate hormonal issues. These sensitivities may trigger inflammation or digestive disturbances, further disrupting hormonal harmony. In this section, we'll explore how to identify and manage these sensitivities within the context of your diet:

Common Food Sensitivities: We'll provide insights into common food sensitivities, such as gluten, dairy, and soy, and explain how they can impact hormonal health. You'll learn how to recognize signs of sensitivity and explore alternatives that support your diet.

Elimination Diets: If you suspect food sensitivities are affecting your hormones, we'll guide you through the process of elimination diets. These structured diets can help you pinpoint problematic foods and alleviate symptoms.

Allergies and Anaphylaxis: For women with food allergies, safety is paramount. We'll discuss strategies for managing severe allergies while maintaining a balanced diet.

## Tracking Progress

As you embark on your personalized Hormonal Balance Diet journey, keeping a journal of your dietary choices and their effects on your hormonal symptoms is a valuable tool. Tracking your progress empowers you to make data-driven adjustments to your diet and assess the effectiveness of your personalized plan:

Symptom Diary: We'll teach you how to maintain a symptom diary to record changes in your energy levels, mood, menstrual cycle, and other relevant indicators of hormonal health. Over time, this diary becomes a valuable reference for understanding how your diet affects your well-being.

Food Journal: Keeping a detailed food journal allows you to monitor your daily nutritional intake. By reviewing this journal alongside your symptom diary, you can identify patterns and make informed adjustments.

Consulting with Experts: If you're unsure about the data you're collecting or need assistance interpreting it, consider consulting with a registered dietitian or healthcare professional. They can provide insights and recommendations based on your progress tracking.

## Planning Your Meals for Hormonal Health

Planning your meals with hormonal health in mind is a crucial aspect of the Hormonal Balance Diet. In this section, you'll receive practical guidance on creating balanced and nutritious meals that support your hormonal goals:

- Sample Meal Plans: We'll provide sample meal plans that align with the Hormonal Balance Diet principles. These plans cater to different dietary preferences and goals, offering inspiration for your own meal planning.

- Recipe Ideas: Discover delicious and hormone-friendly recipes that make adhering to the diet enjoyable. We'll cover breakfast, lunch, dinner, and snacks, showcasing the variety and flavor that can be part of your hormonal balance journey.

- Eating Out and Social Situations: Maintaining your Hormonal Balance Diet in social settings and restaurants can be challenging. We'll share tips on making informed choices when dining out and navigating social gatherings while staying true to your health goals.

# CHAPTER 4

## DETOXIFYING YOUR BODY AND ENVIRONMENT

In this chapter, we delve into the critical topic of detoxification and its pivotal role in achieving hormonal balance. This chapter is a crucial part of the Hormonal Balance Diet for Women, as it provides valuable insights into how we can effectively support our bodies in removing harmful toxins and reducing exposure to endocrine disruptors.

Detoxification is not merely a trendy buzzword; it's a fundamental process that our bodies rely on to maintain health and hormonal equilibrium. When our systems become overwhelmed with toxins from our environment, diet, and lifestyle, it can lead to hormonal imbalances that manifest as a range of troubling symptoms. In this chapter, we explore the significance of detoxification for hormonal balance and provide practical guidance on incorporating detoxifying foods, practices, and habits into your daily life.

Now, let's delve into the subheadings of this Chapterr, each offering comprehensive insights into detoxification and its profound impact on your hormonal well-being.

## The Importance of Detoxification for Hormonal Balance

Detoxification, often referred to as "detox," is not a fleeting health trend but rather a fundamental and intricate physiological process that our bodies rely on for maintaining optimal health and hormonal equilibrium. To truly grasp the significance of detoxification in the context of women's health and hormonal balance, it is imperative to explore the complexities of this process and the profound impact it can have on our overall well-being.

Our bodies are marvels of biological engineering, equipped with an array of mechanisms designed to identify, neutralize, and eliminate harmful substances—effectively functioning as a self-cleaning system. These mechanisms are critical for ensuring that our internal systems operate smoothly and efficiently. However, the modern world has presented us with unprecedented challenges in the form of environmental pollutants, toxins in our food, and chemicals in personal care products. These substances pose a constant threat to our health, particularly our hormonal balance.

In this section, we embark on a comprehensive exploration of the intricate connection between detoxification and hormonal balance. We will delve into the following aspects:

**The Detoxification Process: A Biological Necessity**

Before we delve into the impact of toxins on hormonal balance, it's essential to understand the mechanics of detoxification. Our bodies employ various organs and systems, primarily the liver, kidneys, and lymphatic system, to eliminate toxins and waste products. This process involves a series of complex biochemical reactions that transform harmful substances into less toxic or water-soluble compounds that can be safely excreted through urine, sweat, or feces.

Detoxification is not an optional health practice but a fundamental biological necessity. Without it, our bodies would be overwhelmed by the constant onslaught of toxins from our environment and diet. The liver, for example, plays a central role in detoxification by filtering and neutralizing toxins, ensuring that they do not accumulate to harmful levels in our bloodstream.

**Toxins and Hormonal Imbalance: A Disruptive Connection**

Now, let's explore why detoxification is crucial for hormonal balance. Hormones are intricate chemical messengers that regulate nearly every aspect of our physiology, from our metabolism to our mood. They orchestrate complex processes such as the menstrual cycle, pregnancy, and menopause, making hormonal balance indispensable for women's health.

Toxic substances that infiltrate our bodies can interfere with the delicate symphony of hormone production, regulation, and signaling. The endocrine system, responsible for hormone production, relies on intricate feedback loops to maintain equilibrium. When toxins disrupt these feedback loops, chaos ensues, potentially resulting in a wide range of hormonal imbalances.

## Impact on Menstrual Cycles: More Than Just a Monthly Inconvenience

One of the most noticeable effects of hormonal disruption caused by toxins is irregular menstrual cycles. The menstrual cycle is a highly coordinated dance of hormones, with estrogen and progesterone playing leading roles. When toxins disrupt this delicate balance, it can lead to irregular periods, heavy bleeding, or even missed cycles.

Furthermore, the symptoms of hormonal imbalance extend beyond the physical realm, often manifesting as mood swings, irritability, and emotional instability. Many women have experienced the emotional rollercoaster that accompanies hormonal fluctuations, and toxins can exacerbate these mood swings by disrupting the finely tuned hormonal feedback systems.

## Fertility Challenges: A Consequence of Toxin Exposure

The impact of toxins on hormonal balance goes beyond the monthly menstrual cycle. For women seeking to conceive, hormonal disruptions can pose significant challenges. Fertility relies on the precise orchestration of hormones to ensure ovulation, implantation, and a healthy pregnancy. When toxins interfere with this delicate process, it can lead to difficulties in conceiving or maintaining a pregnancy.

Endocrine-disrupting chemicals found in common household items and environmental pollutants have been linked to fertility issues, including polycystic ovary syndrome (PCOS) and ovulatory disorders. Understanding the role of detoxification in mitigating these risks is crucial for women planning to start a family.

**Specific Hormones in the Spotlight: Estrogen and Progesterone**

To fully grasp the impact of toxins on hormonal balance, it's essential to focus on specific hormones. Estrogen and progesterone, in particular, are central players in the intricate web of hormonal regulation, making them prime targets for disruption by toxins.

Estrogen dominance, a condition where estrogen levels outweigh progesterone levels, is a common consequence of hormonal disruption. This imbalance can lead to symptoms such as heavy periods, breast tenderness, and mood swings. Toxins, often referred to as "xenoestrogens," can mimic the effects of estrogen in the body, further exacerbating estrogen dominance.

On the other hand, progesterone, crucial for maintaining a healthy pregnancy and regulating the menstrual cycle, can also be impacted by toxins. A disrupted balance between estrogen and progesterone can result in anovulation (lack of ovulation), irregular cycles, and difficulties in achieving and maintaining pregnancy.

## Foods and Practices That Support Detoxification

In the quest for hormonal balance and overall well-being, detoxification emerges as a fundamental pillar. While the term "detox" often conjures images of extreme cleanses or deprivation, the reality is quite different. Detoxification is not about punishing your body; it's about nourishing it with the right foods and adopting practices that promote optimal detox function. In this section, we'll embark on a journey into the practical aspects of detoxifying your body through diet and daily routines, demonstrating that detoxification can be a rewarding and enjoyable process.

### The Role of Detoxification in Hormonal Balance

Before we delve into the specific foods and practices that support detoxification, it's crucial to understand why this process is so pivotal for hormonal balance. Our modern world exposes us to an array of toxins and pollutants, from the air we breathe to the food we eat and the products we use. These toxins can disrupt our endocrine system, which regulates hormones, leading to imbalances that manifest as a wide range of health issues.

Hormones, such as estrogen and progesterone, play intricate roles in the female body, influencing menstrual cycles, mood, fertility, and more. When toxins accumulate, they can interfere with hormone production, metabolism, and elimination, throwing these delicate systems out of whack. The result? Irregular menstrual cycles, mood swings, weight gain, and other distressing symptoms.

Detoxification acts as the body's natural defense mechanism against this onslaught of toxins. It involves processes that neutralize and eliminate harmful substances, allowing the body to return to a state of equilibrium. By supporting detoxification, we not only alleviate the burden on our hormonal system but also enhance its functioning, leading to improved well-being.

**The Power of Detoxifying Foods**

One of the most effective ways to support your body's detoxification processes is through your diet. The foods you consume can either burden or bolster your detox organs, with the liver taking center stage. The liver is your body's primary detoxification powerhouse, responsible for processing and eliminating toxins.

Incorporating detoxifying foods into your daily meals can make a significant difference in how efficiently your body detoxifies. Let's explore some of these foods and their roles:

1. Leafy Greens: Leafy green vegetables like spinach, kale, and chard are rich in chlorophyll, a natural detoxifier. Chlorophyll aids in the removal of toxins from the bloodstream, making these greens valuable additions to your diet. You can enjoy them in salads, smoothies, or sautéed as a side dish.

2. Cruciferous Vegetables: Broccoli, cauliflower, Brussels sprouts, and cabbage belong to the cruciferous vegetable family, known for their detoxifying properties. They contain compounds called glucosinolates, which support the liver in detoxifying harmful substances. Roasting or steaming these veggies can bring out their delicious flavors.

3. Antioxidant-Rich Berries: Berries such as blueberries, strawberries, and raspberries are packed with antioxidants that combat oxidative stress and reduce inflammation. They also support the liver's detoxification processes. Enjoy them as snacks, in yogurt, or as toppings for oatmeal.

4. Citrus Fruits: Lemons, limes, oranges, and grapefruits are citrus fruits rich in vitamin C, which stimulates the production of glutathione, a potent antioxidant crucial for detoxification. Start your day with warm water and lemon to kickstart your detox routine.

5. Garlic and Onions: These aromatic vegetables contain sulfur compounds that enhance the liver's detoxifying abilities. They can be incorporated into various savory dishes for added flavor and health benefits.

6. Turmeric: Known for its anti-inflammatory properties, turmeric contains curcumin, a compound that supports liver detoxification. Try adding turmeric to curries, soups, or golden milk.

7. Nuts and Seeds: Walnuts, almonds, chia seeds, and flaxseeds are rich in fiber and omega-3 fatty acids, both of which aid in toxin elimination. They make excellent additions to your breakfast or snacks.

**Practices That Enhance Detoxification**

Detoxification goes beyond what's on your plate. It involves adopting practices that promote the body's self-cleansing mechanisms. Here are some key practices to consider:

1. Intermittent Fasting: Intermittent fasting is an eating pattern that alternates between periods of eating and fasting. This approach can enhance autophagy, the cellular self-cleaning process. By giving your body a break from constant digestion, you allow it to focus on detoxifying and repairing

cells. There are various methods of intermittent fasting, so you can choose one that suits your lifestyle.

2. Staying Hydrated: Proper hydration is essential for the elimination of toxins through urine and sweat. Drinking an adequate amount of water helps the body flush out waste products efficiently. You can also enhance your hydration with herbal teas and infused water for added detox benefits.

3. Regular Exercise: Exercise promotes circulation, which supports the delivery of nutrients to cells and the removal of waste products. It also stimulates the lymphatic system, a key player in detoxification. Incorporate both cardiovascular and strength-training exercises into your routine for optimal results.

4. Stress Reduction Techniques: Chronic stress can hinder detoxification processes. Practices like yoga, meditation, and deep breathing exercises help reduce stress and promote relaxation, allowing your body to focus on detoxifying.

5. Sauna and Sweating: Saunas and hot baths induce sweating, which is another natural way for the body to eliminate toxins. Regular sauna sessions can be a valuable addition to your detox regimen.

6. Quality Sleep: Sleep is when your body undergoes significant repair and detoxification. Aim for seven to nine hours of quality sleep each night to support these essential processes.

## Reducing Exposure to Endocrine Disruptors

In today's modern world, our homes and environments are not the safe havens they once were. Hidden within our daily lives are insidious culprits known as endocrine disruptors—chemicals that have the capacity to impersonate or interfere with our hormonal systems. The consequences of this silent invasion are far-reaching, as they can trigger hormonal imbalances, setting the stage for a cascade of health issues.

Endocrine disruptors are stealthy foes, lurking in various aspects of our lives. To take control of your hormonal health, it's essential to first recognize the common sources of these disruptors:

Plastics: Many plastics contain chemicals like bisphenol-A (BPA) and phthalates that can leach into food, drinks, and even the air. These chemicals can mimic estrogen in the body, potentially leading to hormonal imbalances.

Personal Care Products: Your daily beauty and skincare routines may unknowingly expose you to endocrine disruptors. Ingredients like parabens and fragrance chemicals can interfere with hormone regulation.

Pesticides: Conventionally grown fruits and vegetables often harbor pesticide residues that act as endocrine disruptors when consumed. Washing produce may not be sufficient to eliminate these toxins entirely.

Household Products: Household cleaners, air fresheners, and even some furniture can contain chemicals that disrupt hormonal function. These items release toxins into the air you breathe, affecting your overall well-being.

**Minimizing Exposure: Practical Steps**

Now that we've unveiled the sources of endocrine disruptors, let's explore practical steps to minimize your exposure and protect your hormonal balance:

Choose Hormone-Friendly Household Products: Opt for cleaning products and personal care items labeled as "fragrance-free" or "phthalate-free." Consider natural alternatives like vinegar and baking soda for cleaning.

Go Organic: Whenever possible, choose organic foods, especially for items known as the "Dirty Dozen." These are fruits and vegetables that tend to have higher pesticide residues. By choosing organic, you reduce your exposure to pesticide-based endocrine disruptors.

Mindful Food Storage: Avoid storing food in plastic containers or heating food in plastic containers in the microwave. Instead, opt for glass or stainless steel containers.

Natural Beauty: Look for cosmetics and skincare products made with natural ingredients. Read labels carefully, and consider products labeled "clean" or "green."

Ventilation: Ensure proper ventilation in your home to reduce indoor air pollution from household items. Opening windows and using air purifiers can help.

Educate and Advocate: Stay informed about environmental issues and support regulations that limit the use of harmful chemicals. As consumers, our choices and voices can influence industry practices.

By taking these practical steps, you empower yourself to reduce your exposure to endocrine disruptors, safeguarding your hormonal health. This section is not just about identifying the threats but providing you with actionable strategies to reclaim control over your environment and, in turn, your well-being. As you implement these changes, you'll move one step closer to achieving hormonal balance and enjoying the lasting benefits of a healthier, harmonious life.

# CHAPTER 5

## RECIPES FOR HORMONAL BALANCE AND MEAL PLAN

**Breakfast recipes to kickstart your day**

### 1. Hormone-Balancing Smoothie Bowl

**Ingredients:**

1 cup mixed berries (strawberries, blueberries, raspberries)

1/2 banana

1/2 cup Greek yogurt

1 tbsp ground flaxseeds

1 tsp honey

1/4 cup granola

**Instructions:**

Blend mixed berries, banana, Greek yogurt, and flaxseeds until smooth.

Pour into a bowl, drizzle with honey, and sprinkle with granola.

**Nutritional Information (approx.):**

Calories: 350

Protein: 12g

Fiber: 7g

Healthy fats: 5g

## 2. Spinach and Mushroom Omelette

**Ingredients:**

2 eggs

1 cup fresh spinach leaves

1/2 cup sliced mushrooms

1/4 cup diced onions

Salt and pepper to taste

**Instructions:**

Whisk eggs in a bowl and season with salt and pepper.

Sauté spinach, mushrooms, and onions in a non-stick pan until wilted.

Pour whisked eggs over the veggies and cook until set. Fold in half.

**Nutritional Information (approx.):**

Calories: 250

Protein: 16g

Fiber: 3g

Healthy fats: 10g

## 3. Chia Seed Pudding

**Ingredients:**

2 tbsp chia seeds

1 cup almond milk (unsweetened)

1/2 tsp vanilla extract

1/2 cup mixed berries

1 tsp honey (optional)

**Instructions:**

Mix chia seeds, almond milk, and vanilla extract in a jar.

Refrigerate for at least 2 hours or overnight.

Top with mixed berries and drizzle with honey.

**Nutritional Information (approx.):**

Calories: 180

Protein: 5g

Fiber: 10g

Healthy fats: 8g

## 4. Avocado Toast with Poached Egg

**Ingredients:**

1 slice whole-grain bread

1/2 ripe avocado, mashed

1 poached egg

Salt, pepper, and red pepper flakes to taste

**Instructions:**

Toast the bread and spread mashed avocado on top.

Place a poached egg on the avocado.

Season with salt, pepper, and red pepper flakes.

**Nutritional Information (approx.):**

Calories: 250

Protein: 10g

Fiber: 7g

Healthy fats: 15g

## 5. Greek Yogurt Parfait

**Ingredients:**

1 cup Greek yogurt

1/2 cup mixed berries

1 tbsp honey

2 tbsp granola

**Instructions:**

Layer Greek yogurt, mixed berries, and granola in a glass.

Drizzle with honey.

**Nutritional Information (approx.):**

Calories: 280

Protein: 14g

Fiber: 4g

Healthy fats: 5g

## 6. Quinoa Breakfast Bowl

**Ingredients:**

1/2 cup cooked quinoa

1/4 cup sliced almonds

1/2 cup diced mango

1/2 tsp cinnamon

1 tsp honey

**Instructions:**

Combine cooked quinoa, sliced almonds, and diced mango in a bowl.

Sprinkle with cinnamon and drizzle with honey.

**Nutritional Information (approx.):**

Calories: 280

Protein: 6g

Fiber: 6g

Healthy fats: 5g

## 7. Almond Butter Banana Toast

**Ingredients:**

1 slice whole-grain bread

2 tbsp almond butter

1/2 banana, sliced

**Instructions:**

Toast the bread and spread almond butter on top.

Arrange banana slices on the almond butter.

**Nutritional Information (approx.):**

Calories: 280

Protein: 7g

Fiber: 6g

Healthy fats: 12g

## 8. Berry Nut Oatmeal

**Ingredients:**

1/2 cup rolled oats

1 cup almond milk (unsweetened)

1/2 cup mixed berries

1 tbsp chopped nuts (almonds, walnuts)

1 tsp honey

**Instructions:**

Cook rolled oats with almond milk until creamy.

Top with mixed berries, chopped nuts, and honey.

**Nutritional Information (approx.):**

Calories: 320

Protein: 8g

Fiber: 7g

Healthy fats: 7g

## 9. Sweet Potato Breakfast Hash

**Ingredients:**

1 small sweet potato, diced

1/4 cup diced bell peppers

1/4 cup diced onions

1/4 cup black beans (cooked)

1/2 tsp cumin

Salt and pepper to taste

**Instructions:**

Sauté sweet potatoes, bell peppers, and onions until tender.

Add black beans, cumin, salt, and pepper. Cook for another 2 minutes.

**Nutritional Information (approx.):**

Calories: 290

Protein: 9g

Fiber: 8g

Healthy fats: 2g

**10. Smoked Salmon and Avocado Wrap**

**Ingredients:** 1 whole-grain tortilla

2 oz smoked salmon

1/4 avocado, sliced

1/4 cup cucumber slices

1 tsp Greek yogurt

**Instructions:**

1. Lay the tortilla flat and layer with smoked salmon, avocado, and cucumber.

2. Drizzle with Greek yogurt and roll into a wrap.

**Nutritional Information (approx.):**

Calories: 290

Protein: 15g

Fiber: 6g

Healthy fats: 14g

## 11. Blueberry Almond Protein Pancakes

**- Ingredients:**

- 1/2 cup almond flour

- 2 eggs

- 1/4 cup almond milk (unsweetened)

- 1/4 cup blueberries

- 1/2 tsp baking powder

- 1 tsp honey

**- Instructions:**

1. Mix almond flour, eggs, almond milk, and baking powder until smooth.

2. Fold in blueberries.

3. Cook pancakes on a non-stick pan until golden brown.

4. Drizzle with honey.

**- Nutritional Information (approx.):**

- Calories: 330

- Protein: 11g

- Fiber: 4g

- Healthy fats: 23g

## 12. Green Shakshuka

**Ingredients:** 2 eggs

- 1 cup spinach

- 1/4 cup diced tomatoes

- 1/4 cup diced onions

- 1/2 tsp cumin

- Salt and pepper to taste

**Instructions:**

1. Sauté spinach, tomatoes, and onions in a pan until wilted.

2. Create two wells in the mixture and crack eggs into them.

3. Sprinkle with cumin, salt, and pepper.

4. Cover and cook until eggs are done to your liking.

**Nutritional Information (approx.):**

- Calories: 280

- Protein: 14g

- Fiber: 6g

- Healthy fats: 8g

## 13. Almond Berry Breakfast Quinoa

**Ingredients:** 1/2 cup cooked quinoa

- 1/4 cup sliced almonds

- 1/2 cup mixed berries

- 1 tsp honey

**Instructions:**

1. Combine cooked quinoa, sliced almonds, and mixed berries in a bowl.

2. Drizzle with honey.

**Nutritional Information (approx.):**

- Calories: 280

- Protein: 8g

- Fiber: 5g

- Healthy fats: 8g

## 14. Turmeric Scrambled Tofu

**Ingredients:**

- 1/2 block firm tofu, crumbled

- 1/4 cup diced bell peppers

- 1/4 cup diced onions

- 1/2 tsp turmeric

- Salt and pepper to taste

**Instructions:**

1. Sauté crumbled tofu, bell peppers, and onions until heated through.

2. Sprinkle with turmeric, salt, and pepper.

**Nutritional Information (approx.):**

- Calories: 270

- Protein: 14g

- Fiber: 4g

- Healthy fats: 12g

## 15. Peanut Butter Banana Overnight Oats

**Ingredients:**

- 1/2 cup rolled oats

- 1 cup almond milk (unsweetened)

- 2 tbsp peanut butter

- 1/2 banana, sliced

**Instructions:**

1. Mix rolled oats, almond milk, and peanut butter in a jar.

2. Refrigerate overnight.

3. Top with banana slices in the morning.

**Nutritional Information (approx.):**

- Calories: 340

- Protein: 11g

- Fiber: 8g

- Healthy fats: 14g

## 16. Berry and Almond Butter Toast

**Ingredients:**

- 1 slice whole-grain bread

- 2 tbsp almond butter

- 1/2 cup mixed berries

- 1 tsp honey

**Instructions:**

1. Toast the bread and spread almond butter on top.

2. Arrange mixed berries on the almond butter.

3. Drizzle with honey.

**Nutritional Information (approx.):**

- Calories: 290

- Protein: 8g

- Fiber: 6g

- Healthy fats: 14g

## 17. Pumpkin Spice Chia Pudding

**Ingredients:**

- 2 tbsp chia seeds

- 1 cup almond milk (unsweetened)

- 1/4 cup canned pumpkin puree

- 1/2 tsp pumpkin spice

- 1 tsp maple syrup (optional)

**Instructions:**

1. Mix chia seeds, almond milk, pumpkin puree, and pumpkin spice in a jar.

2. Refrigerate for at least 2 hours or overnight.

3. Drizzle with maple syrup if desired.

**Nutritional Information (approx.):**

- Calories: 200

- Protein: 6g

- Fiber: 9g

- Healthy fats: 9g

## 18. Veggie and Quinoa Breakfast Bowl

**Ingredients:**

- 1/2 cup cooked quinoa

- 1/4 cup diced tomatoes

- 1/4 cup diced bell peppers

- 1/4 cup diced onions

- 1/4 cup black beans (cooked)

- 1/2 tsp cumin

- Salt and pepper to taste

**Instructions:**

1. Sauté tomatoes, bell peppers, and onions until tender.

2. Add cooked quinoa, black beans, cumin, salt, and pepper. Cook for another 2 minutes.

**Nutritional Information (approx.):**

- Calories: 290

- Protein: 9g

- Fiber: 6g

- Healthy fats: 2g

## 19. Apple Cinnamon Breakfast Quinoa

**Ingredients:**

- 1/2 cup cooked quinoa

- 1/2 apple, diced

- 1/4 tsp cinnamon

- 1 tsp honey

**Instructions:**

1. Combine cooked quinoa, diced apple, and cinnamon in a bowl.

2. Drizzle with honey.

**Nutritional Information (approx.):**

- Calories: 250

- Protein: 6g

- Fiber: 5g

- Healthy fats: 1g

## 20. Veggie Omelette Wrap

- Ingredients:

- 2 eggs

- 1/4 cup diced bell peppers

- 1/4 cup diced onions

- 1/4 cup spinach leaves

- Salt and pepper to taste

- 1 whole-grain tortilla

**Instructions:**

1. Whisk eggs in a bowl and season with salt and pepper.

2. Sauté bell peppers, onions, and spinach until wilted.

3. Pour whisked eggs over the veggies and cook until set. Roll into a wrap using a whole-grain tortilla.

**Nutritional Information (approx.):**

- Calories: 300

- Protein: 15g

- Fiber: 5g

- Healthy fats: 10g

## 1. Quinoa and Chickpea Salad

**Ingredients:**

1 cup cooked quinoa

1/2 cup chickpeas (canned or cooked)

Cherry tomatoes

Cucumber

Red onion

Fresh parsley

Lemon juice

Olive oil

Salt and pepper

**Instructions:**

In a bowl, combine cooked quinoa and chickpeas.

Add cherry tomatoes, cucumber, and red onion, all diced.

Sprinkle with fresh parsley.

Drizzle with lemon juice and olive oil.

Season with salt and pepper to taste.

**Nutritional Information (per serving):**

Calories: 350

Protein: 12g

Fiber: 8g

Healthy fats: 10g

## 2. Salmon and Avocado Wrap

**Ingredients:**

Whole-grain tortilla

Grilled salmon fillet

Sliced avocado

Spinach leaves

Greek yogurt

Dill

Lemon zest

**Instructions:**

Lay a whole-grain tortilla flat.

Place grilled salmon, sliced avocado, and spinach leaves on the tortilla.

Mix Greek yogurt with dill and lemon zest, then spread it on top.

Roll the tortilla into a wrap and slice in half.

**Nutritional Information (per serving):**

Calories: 400

Protein: 25g

Fiber: 7g

Healthy fats: 20g

# 3. Lentil and Vegetable Soup

## Ingredients:

Red lentils

Carrots

Celery

Onion

Garlic

Vegetable broth

Turmeric

Cumin

Coriander

Spinach

## Instructions:

Sauté onions, garlic, carrots, and celery in a pot.

Add red lentils and vegetable broth.

Season with turmeric, cumin, and coriander.

Simmer until lentils are tender.

Stir in fresh spinach before serving.

## Nutritional Information (per serving):

Calories: 280

Protein: 15g

Fiber: 10g

Healthy fats: 2g

## 4. Quinoa and Black Bean Bowl

**Ingredients:**

Cooked quinoa

Black beans (canned or cooked)

Bell peppers

Corn kernels

Avocado

Cilantro

Lime juice

Olive oil

Chili powder

**Instructions:**

Combine cooked quinoa and black beans in a bowl.

Add diced bell peppers, corn kernels, and avocado.

Toss with cilantro, lime juice, olive oil, and a dash of chili powder.

**Nutritional Information (per serving):**

Calories: 380

Protein: 12g

Fiber: 11g

Healthy fats: 15g

## 5. Greek Salad with Grilled Chicken

**Ingredients:**

Grilled chicken breast

Cucumber

Cherry tomatoes

Red onion

Kalamata olives

Feta cheese

Romaine lettuce

Greek dressing

**Instructions:**

Slice grilled chicken breast.

Combine with cucumber, cherry tomatoes, red onion, Kalamata olives, and feta cheese.

Serve over a bed of romaine lettuce.

Drizzle with Greek dressing.

**Nutritional Information (per serving):**

Calories: 380

Protein: 30g

Fiber: 4g

Healthy fats: 16g

## 6. Sweet Potato and Chickpea Bowl

**Ingredients:**

Roasted sweet potato cubes

Chickpeas (canned or cooked)

Baby spinach

Red bell pepper

Red onion

Tahini dressing

**Instructions:**

Combine roasted sweet potato cubes and chickpeas in a bowl.

Add baby spinach, diced red bell pepper, and thinly sliced red onion.

Drizzle with tahini dressing.

**Nutritional Information (per serving):**

Calories: 380

Protein: 12g

Fiber: 10g

Healthy fats: 14g

## 7. Tuna and White Bean Salad

**Ingredients:**

Canned tuna in water

White beans (canned or cooked)

Cherry tomatoes

Red onion

Kalamata olives

Fresh basil

Olive oil and balsamic vinegar

**Instructions:**

Drain canned tuna and white beans.

Mix with halved cherry tomatoes, thinly sliced red onion, Kalamata olives, and fresh basil leaves.

Drizzle with olive oil and balsamic vinegar.

**Nutritional Information (per serving):**

Calories: 340

Protein: 25g

Fiber: 7g

Healthy fats: 15g

## 8. Spinach and Quinoa Stuffed Bell Peppers

**Ingredients:**

Bell peppers (various colors)

Cooked quinoa

Baby spinach

Cherry tomatoes

Feta cheese

Olive oil

Garlic powder

Italian seasoning

**Instructions:**

Cut the tops off bell peppers and remove seeds.

Stuff with a mixture of cooked quinoa, baby spinach, halved cherry tomatoes, and crumbled feta cheese.

Drizzle with olive oil and sprinkle with garlic powder and Italian seasoning.

Bake until peppers are tender.

**Nutritional Information (per serving):**

Calories: 320

Protein: 10g

Fiber: 8g

Healthy fats: 12g

## 9. Asian-Inspired Tofu Salad

**Ingredients:** Baked or pan-fried tofu cubes

Mixed greens

Edamame

Shredded carrots

Sliced cucumber

Sesame ginger dressing

**Instructions:**

Combine baked or pan-fried tofu cubes with mixed greens, edamame, shredded carrots, and sliced cucumber.

Drizzle with sesame ginger dressing.

**Nutritional Information (per serving):**

Calories: 360

Protein: 16g

Fiber: 10g

Healthy fats: 14g

## 10. Mediterranean Quinoa Bowl

**Ingredients:**

Cooked quinoa

Grilled chicken or chickpeas

Cucumber

Cherry tomatoes

Red onion

Kalamata olives

Feta cheese

Tzatziki sauce

**Instructions:** Layer cooked quinoa with grilled chicken or chickpeas, diced cucumber, halved cherry tomatoes, thinly sliced red onion, Kalamata olives, and crumbled feta cheese.

Drizzle with tzatziki sauce.

**Nutritional Information (per serving):**

Calories: 390

Protein: 24g

Fiber: 7g

Healthy fats: 16g

## 11. Spinach and Mushroom Quiche

**Ingredients:**

Whole-grain pie crust

Eggs

Baby spinach

Sliced mushrooms

Onion

Low-fat milk

Swiss cheese

Nutmeg

Salt and pepper

**Instructions:**

Preheat the oven and bake the pie crust until lightly browned.

Sauté sliced mushrooms and onions until tender.

In a bowl, whisk together eggs, low-fat milk, nutmeg, salt, and pepper.

Layer baby spinach, sautéed mushrooms, and Swiss cheese in the pie crust.

Pour the egg mixture over the top.

Bake until the quiche is set and golden brown.

**Nutritional Information (per serving):**

Calories: 340

Protein: 15g

Fiber: 4g

Healthy fats: 18g

## 12. Turkey and Avocado Wrap

**Ingredients:**

Whole-grain tortilla

Sliced turkey breast

Sliced avocado

Baby spinach

Hummus

Red bell pepper strips

**Instructions:**

Lay a whole-grain tortilla flat.

Place sliced turkey breast, sliced avocado, baby spinach, and red bell pepper strips on the tortilla.

Spread a thin layer of hummus.

Roll the tortilla into a wrap and slice in half.

**Nutritional Information (per serving):**

Calories: 320

Protein: 25g

Fiber: 7g

Healthy fats: 15g

## 13. Quinoa and Roasted Vegetable Bowl

**Ingredients:**

Cooked quinoa

Roasted sweet potatoes, broccoli, and red bell peppers

Chickpeas (canned or cooked)

Tahini dressing

**Instructions:**

Combine cooked quinoa, roasted vegetables, and chickpeas in a bowl.

Drizzle with tahini dressing.

**Nutritional Information (per serving):**

Calories: 360

Protein: 12g

Fiber: 10g

Healthy fats: 14g

## 14. Caprese Salad with Grilled Chicken

**Ingredients:**

Grilled chicken breast

Fresh mozzarella cheese

Ripe tomatoes

Fresh basil leaves

Balsamic glaze

Olive oil

Salt and pepper

**Instructions:**

Slice grilled chicken breast, fresh mozzarella cheese, and ripe tomatoes.

Arrange on a plate with fresh basil leaves.

Drizzle with balsamic glaze and olive oil.

Season with salt and pepper to taste.

**Nutritional Information (per serving):**

Calories: 380

Protein: 30g

Fiber: 3g

Healthy fats: 18g

## 15. Veggie and Hummus Wrap

**Ingredients:**

Whole-grain tortilla

Hummus

Sliced cucumber

Sliced red bell pepper

Baby spinach

Sliced carrots

**Instructions:**

Lay a whole-grain tortilla flat.

Spread a generous layer of hummus.

Layer sliced cucumber, red bell pepper, baby spinach, and sliced carrots.

Roll the tortilla into a wrap and slice in half.

**Nutritional Information (per serving):**

Calories: 290

Protein: 8g

Fiber: 7g

Healthy fats: 12g

**16. Moroccan Chickpea and Quinoa Salad**

**Ingredients:**

Cooked quinoa

Chickpeas (canned or cooked)

Diced cucumber

Dried apricots

Chopped fresh mint

Lemon vinaigrette

**Instructions:**

Combine cooked quinoa, chickpeas, diced cucumber, dried apricots, and chopped fresh mint in a bowl.

Drizzle with lemon vinaigrette.

**Nutritional Information (per serving):**

Calories: 370

Protein: 12g

Fiber: 9g

Healthy fats: 15g

## 17. Shrimp and Avocado Salad

**Ingredients:**

Grilled shrimp

Sliced avocado

Mixed greens

Cherry tomatoes

Red onion

Cilantro

Lime vinaigrette

**Instructions:**

Combine grilled shrimp, sliced avocado, mixed greens, halved cherry tomatoes, thinly sliced red onion, and cilantro.

Drizzle with lime vinaigrette.

**Nutritional Information (per serving):**

Calories: 350

Protein: 22g

Fiber: 7g

Healthy fats: 18g

## 18. Roasted Vegetable and Quinoa Wrap

**Ingredients:** Whole-grain tortilla

Roasted zucchini, eggplant, and red bell peppers

Cooked quinoa

Hummus

**Instructions:**

Lay a whole-grain tortilla flat.

Spread a layer of hummus.

Layer roasted zucchini, eggplant, and red bell peppers, along with cooked quinoa.

Roll the tortilla into a wrap and slice in half.

**Nutritional Information (per serving):**

Calories: 320

Protein: 10g

Fiber: 9g

Healthy fats: 14g

## 19. Tofu and Broccoli Stir-Fry

**Ingredients:**

Tofu cubes

Broccoli florets

Red bell pepper strips

Sliced carrots

Garlic ginger stir-fry sauce

**Instructions:**

Stir-fry tofu cubes until lightly browned.

Add broccoli florets, red bell pepper strips, and sliced carrots.

Stir in garlic ginger stir-fry sauce and cook until vegetables are tender.

**Nutritional Information (per serving):**

Calories: 350

Protein: 15g

Fiber: 8g

Healthy fats: 10g

## 20. Mediterranean Couscous Salad

**Ingredients:**

Cooked couscous

Diced cucumbers

Cherry tomatoes

Red onion

Kalamata olives

Fresh parsley

Lemon vinaigrette

**Instructions:**

Combine cooked couscous, diced cucumbers, halved cherry tomatoes, diced red onion, Kalamata olives, and fresh parsley in a bowl.

Drizzle with lemon vinaigrette.

**Nutritional Information (per serving):**

Calories: 360

Protein: 8g

Fiber: 4g

Healthy fats: 10g

# Satisfying dinners for overall health

## 1. Grilled Salmon with Asparagus

**Ingredients:**

2 salmon fillets (6 ounces each)

1 bunch of asparagus

2 tablespoons olive oil

1 tablespoon lemon juice

2 cloves garlic, minced

Salt and pepper to taste

**Instructions:**

Preheat the grill.

Brush salmon and asparagus with olive oil.

Season with lemon juice, minced garlic, salt, and pepper.

Grill salmon for 4-5 minutes on each side.

Grill asparagus for 3-4 minutes.

Serve salmon and asparagus together.

**Nutritional Information (per serving):**

Calories: 350 | Protein: 30g | Carbohydrates: 6g | Fat: 22g

## 2. Quinoa and Chickpea Stir-Fry

**Ingredients:** 1 cup quinoa

1 can chickpeas (15 ounces)

Mixed vegetables (1 cup, e.g., bell peppers, broccoli, carrots)

2 tablespoons low-sodium soy sauce

1 teaspoon grated ginger

2 cloves garlic, minced

1 tablespoon sesame oil

**Instructions:**

Cook quinoa according to package instructions.

In a wok, sauté mixed vegetables with ginger and garlic.

Add cooked chickpeas.

Stir in cooked quinoa.

Drizzle with low-sodium soy sauce and sesame oil.

**Nutritional Information (per serving):**

Calories: 400 | Protein: 15g | Carbohydrates: 70g | Fat: 9g

### 3. Lentil and Vegetable Curry

**Ingredients:**

1 cup red lentils

Mixed vegetables (e.g., 1 zucchini, 1 cup spinach, 2 tomatoes)

1 can coconut milk (14 ounces)

2 teaspoons curry powder

1/2 teaspoon turmeric

1/2 teaspoon cumin

2 cloves garlic, minced

**Instructions:**

Cook lentils according to package instructions.

In a pan, sauté mixed vegetables with garlic and spices.

Stir in cooked lentils and coconut milk.

Simmer until vegetables are tender.

**Nutritional Information (per serving):**

Calories: 320 | Protein: 15g | Carbohydrates: 45g | Fat: 10g

## 4. Baked Sweet Potato with Black Beans

**Ingredients:**

2 sweet potatoes

1 can black beans (15 ounces)

1 avocado

1 lime, juiced

Fresh cilantro for garnish

Paprika for sprinkling

**Instructions:**

Bake sweet potatoes until tender.

Heat black beans.

Mash avocado with lime juice and cilantro.

Serve sweet potatoes topped with black beans and avocado mixture. Sprinkle with paprika.

**Nutritional Information (per serving):**

Calories: 320 | Protein: 10g | Carbohydrates: 60g | Fat: 8g

**5. Turkey and Spinach Stuffed Bell Peppers**

**Ingredients:**

4 bell peppers

1/2 pound ground turkey

1 cup spinach

1/2 cup cooked quinoa

1 cup tomato sauce

1/2 onion, chopped

1 teaspoon Italian seasoning

**Instructions:**

Cut the tops off bell peppers and remove seeds.

Brown ground turkey with onion and Italian seasoning.

Add cooked quinoa and spinach.

Stuff bell peppers with the mixture.

Bake with tomato sauce until peppers are tender.

**Nutritional Information (per serving):**

Calories: 350 | Protein: 25g | Carbohydrates: 30g | Fat: 12g

## 6. Veggie and Chickpea Salad

**Ingredients:** Mixed greens (4 cups)

Cherry tomatoes (1 cup)

1 cucumber, sliced

1/2 red onion, thinly sliced

1 can chickpeas (15 ounces)

Feta cheese (optional)

Balsamic vinaigrette dressing

**Instructions:**

Combine mixed greens, cherry tomatoes, cucumber, red onion, and chickpeas.

Top with crumbled feta cheese.

Drizzle with balsamic vinaigrette.

**Nutritional Information (per serving):**

Calories: 300 | Protein: 10g | Carbohydrates: 35g | Fat: 15g

## 7. Broccoli and Almond Stir-Fry

**Ingredients:** Broccoli florets (3 cups)

Sliced almonds (1/4 cup)

2 tablespoons low-sodium soy sauce

1 teaspoon grated ginger

2 cloves garlic, minced

Cooked brown rice (2 cups)

**Instructions:**

Steam broccoli until tender.

In a pan, sauté sliced almonds with ginger and garlic.

Add steamed broccoli.

Serve over cooked brown rice, drizzled with low-sodium soy sauce.

**Nutritional Information (per serving):**

Calories: 280 | Protein: 9g | Carbohydrates: 45g | Fat: 7g

## 8. Grilled Chicken with Brussels Sprouts

**Ingredients:**

2 chicken breasts

Brussels sprouts (2 cups)

2 tablespoons olive oil

Zest of 1 lemon

1 teaspoon dried rosemary

Salt and pepper to taste

**Instructions:**

Marinate chicken in olive oil, lemon zest, rosemary, salt, and pepper.

Grill chicken until cooked through.

Roast Brussels sprouts with olive oil, salt, and pepper.

Serve chicken with roasted Brussels sprouts.

**Nutritional Information (per serving):**

Calories: 320 | Protein: 30g | Carbohydrates: 12g | Fat: 15g

## 9. Spinach and Mushroom Omelette

**Ingredients:**

3 eggs

1 cup spinach

Mushrooms (1/2 cup)

1/4 onion, diced

Cheese (optional)

1 tablespoon olive oil

**Instructions:**

Sauté mushrooms and onion in olive oil.

Whisk eggs and pour into the pan.

Add spinach and cheese (if desired).

Cook until set and fold in half.

**Nutritional Information (per serving):**

Calories: 250 | Protein: 18g | Carbohydrates: 6g | Fat: 16g

## 10. Tofu and Vegetable Stir-Fry

**Ingredients:**

1 block tofu

Broccoli florets (1 cup)

Bell peppers (1 cup)

Snow peas (1 cup)

1/4 cup teriyaki sauce

1 teaspoon grated ginger

2 cloves garlic, minced

Cooked brown rice (2 cups)

**Instructions:**

Cut tofu into cubes and stir-fry with ginger and garlic.

Add broccoli, bell peppers, and snow peas.

Drizzle with teriyaki sauce.

Serve over cooked brown rice.

**Nutritional Information (per serving):**

Calories: 300 | Protein: 15g | Carbohydrates: 45g | Fat: 8g

## 11. Cilantro Lime Shrimp and Quinoa

**Ingredients:**

Shrimp (1/2 pound)

1 cup quinoa

Fresh cilantro

Juice of 2 limes

2 cloves garlic, minced

Paprika

1 avocado

**Instructions:**

Cook quinoa according to package instructions.

Sauté shrimp with minced garlic, paprika, and lime juice.

Stir in chopped cilantro.

Serve over cooked quinoa with avocado slices.

**Nutritional Information (per serving):**

Calories: 320 | Protein: 25g | Carbohydrates: 30g | Fat: 12g

## 12. Butternut Squash and Sage Pasta

**Ingredients:**

Whole wheat pasta (8 ounces)

Butternut squash (1/2 medium)

Sage leaves (8-10 leaves)

2 tablespoons olive oil

Parmesan cheese (optional)

**Instructions:**

Roast butternut squash with sage leaves and olive oil.

Cook whole wheat pasta.

Toss pasta with roasted squash.

Sprinkle with Parmesan cheese if desired.

**Nutritional Information (per serving):**

Calories: 350 | Protein: 10g | Carbohydrates: 65g | Fat: 8g

## 13. Baked Cod with Roasted Vegetables

**Ingredients:**

Cod fillets (2 fillets)

Mixed vegetables (carrots, bell peppers, onions) (2 cups)

2 tablespoons olive oil

Zest of 1 lemon

Fresh dill

Salt and pepper to taste

**Instructions:**

Place cod fillets on a baking sheet.

Toss mixed vegetables with olive oil, lemon juice, dill, salt, and pepper.

Bake cod and vegetables until cooked through.

**Nutritional Information (per serving):**

Calories: 280 | Protein: 25g | Carbohydrates: 20g | Fat: 12g

## 14. Brown Rice and Black Bean Bowl

**Ingredients:**

Brown rice (2 cups)

Black beans (1 can, 15 ounces)

1 avocado

Salsa

Fresh cilantro

Lime wedges

**Instructions:**

Cook brown rice according to package instructions.

Warm black beans.

Assemble bowls with rice, black beans, avocado, salsa, cilantro, and lime wedges.

**Nutritional Information (per serving):**

Calories: 320 | Protein: 10g | Carbohydrates: 55g | Fat: 8g

## 15. Beef and Broccoli Stir-Fry

**Ingredients:** Lean beef strips (1/2 pound)

Broccoli florets (2 cups)

2 tablespoons low-sodium soy sauce

2 teaspoons grated ginger

2 cloves garlic, minced

Cooked brown rice (2 cups)

**Instructions:**

Sauté beef strips with garlic and ginger.

Add broccoli florets and low-sodium soy sauce.

Serve over cooked brown rice.

**Nutritional Information (per serving):**

Calories: 340 | Protein: 25g | Carbohydrates: 45g | Fat: 10g

# 21-Day Sample Meal Plan

**Week 1**

**Day 1:**

Breakfast: Hormone-Boosting Breakfast Smoothie

Lunch: Quinoa and Chickpea Salad with Tahini Dressing

Snack: Greek Yogurt with Honey and Cinnamon

Dinner: Grilled Salmon with Steamed Broccoli and Chia Seeds

**Day 2:**

Breakfast: Avocado Toast with Poached Egg

Lunch: Spinach and Feta Stuffed Bell Peppers

Snack: Almonds

Dinner: Quinoa-Crusted Fish with Asparagus

**Day 3:**

Breakfast: Chia Seed Pudding with Mango

Lunch: Turkey and Avocado Wrap with a Side of Mixed Greens

Snack: Carrot Sticks with Almond Butter

Dinner: Spaghetti Squash with Tomato and Basil Sauce

**Day 4:**

Breakfast: Oatmeal with Berries and Flaxseeds

Lunch: Lentil Soup with a Side Salad

Snack: Sliced Cucumbers with Hummus

Dinner: Stir-Fried Tofu with Broccoli and Brown Rice

**Day 5:**

Breakfast: Greek Yogurt Parfait with Berries

Lunch: Quinoa and Black Bean Bowl with Guacamole

Snack: Apple Slices with Peanut Butter

Dinner: Grilled Shrimp with Quinoa and Roasted Brussels Sprouts

**Day 6:**

Breakfast: Banana Walnut Pancakes (using almond flour)

Lunch: Sweet Potato and Chickpea Curry

Snack: Greek Yogurt with Sliced Kiwi

Dinner: Baked Cod with Lemon and Dill, served with Steamed Asparagus

**Day 7:**

Breakfast: Hormone-Boosting Breakfast Smoothie

Lunch: Leftover Quinoa and Chickpea Salad

Snack: Mixed Berries

Dinner: Baked Chicken Breast with Roasted Vegetables

**Week 2**

**Day 1:**

Breakfast: Greek Yogurt Parfait with Berries

Lunch: Spinach and Feta Stuffed Bell Peppers

Snack: Sliced Cucumbers with Hummus

Dinner: Quinoa-Crusted Fish with Asparagus

**Day 2:**

Breakfast: Chia Seed Pudding with Mango

Lunch: Quinoa and Black Bean Bowl with Guacamole

Snack: Apple Slices with Peanut Butter

Dinner: Grilled Shrimp with Quinoa and Roasted Brussels Sprouts

**Day 3:**

Breakfast: Oatmeal with Berries and Flaxseeds

Lunch: Lentil Soup with a Side Salad

Snack: Mixed Berries

Dinner: Stir-Fried Tofu with Broccoli and Brown Rice

**Day 4:**

Breakfast: Avocado Toast with Poached Egg

Lunch: Sweet Potato and Chickpea Curry

Snack: Greek Yogurt with Sliced Kiwi

Dinner: Baked Cod with Lemon and Dill, served with Steamed Asparagus

**Day 5:**

Breakfast: Banana Walnut Pancakes (using almond flour)

Lunch: Quinoa and Chickpea Salad with Tahini Dressing

Snack: Almonds

Dinner: Spaghetti Squash with Tomato and Basil Sauce

**Day 6:**

Breakfast: Hormone-Boosting Breakfast Smoothie

Lunch: Leftover Quinoa and Chickpea Salad

Snack: Carrot Sticks with Almond Butter

Dinner: Grilled Salmon with Steamed Broccoli and Chia Seeds

**Day 7:**

Breakfast: Chia Seed Pudding with Berries

Lunch: Turkey and Avocado Wrap with a Side of Mixed Greens

Snack: Greek Yogurt with Honey and Cinnamon

Dinner: Baked Chicken Breast with Roasted Vegetables

**Week 3**

**Day 1:**

Breakfast: Hormone-Boosting Breakfast Smoothie

Lunch: Quinoa and Chickpea Salad with Tahini Dressing

Snack: Greek Yogurt with Honey and Berries

Dinner: Grilled Salmon with Asparagus and Quinoa

**Day 2:**

Breakfast: Chia Seed Pudding with Mango and Almonds

Lunch: Spinach and Feta Stuffed Bell Peppers

Snack: Sliced Cucumbers with Hummus

Dinner: Lemon Herb Roasted Chicken with Steamed Broccoli

**Day 3:**

Breakfast: Avocado Toast with Poached Egg

Lunch: Lentil Soup with a Side Salad

Snack: Mixed Berries with a Dollop of Greek Yogurt

Dinner: Tofu and Vegetable Stir-Fry with Brown Rice

**Day 4:**

Breakfast: Greek Yogurt Parfait with Berries and Granola

Lunch: Quinoa and Black Bean Bowl with Guacamole

Snack: Apple Slices with Almond Butter

Dinner: Baked Cod with Lemon and Dill, served with Roasted Brussels Sprouts

**Day 5:**

Breakfast: Oatmeal with Berries and Flaxseeds

Lunch: Sweet Potato and Chickpea Curry

Snack: Sliced Kiwi with a Sprinkle of Chia Seeds

Dinner: Grilled Shrimp with Quinoa and Steamed Asparagus

**Day 6:**

Breakfast: Banana Walnut Pancakes (using almond flour)

Lunch: Quinoa and Chickpea Salad with Tahini Dressing

Snack: Mixed Nuts

Dinner: Spaghetti Squash with Tomato and Basil Sauce

**Day 7:**

Breakfast: Hormone-Boosting Breakfast Smoothie

Lunch: Turkey and Avocado Wrap with a Side of Mixed Greens

Snack: Carrot Sticks with Hummus

Dinner: Baked Chicken Breast with Roasted Vegetables

# CHAPTER 6

## SUPPLEMENTATION AND HORMONAL HEALTH

In this Chapter of "Hormonal Balance Diet for Women," we delve into the crucial topic of supplementation and its role in supporting hormonal health. As we navigate this chapter, we'll explore the diverse landscape of supplements, their effectiveness in promoting hormonal balance, and the critical factors to consider when incorporating them into your wellness routine. Understanding the nuances of supplements, dosages, and quality is paramount, as is learning how to seamlessly integrate these supplements into your daily diet for maximum impact.

Now, let's embark on this informative journey, beginning with a comprehensive discussion of the supplements that hold promise in the realm of hormonal balance.

### Supplements for Hormonal Balance: What Works?

The quest for hormonal balance often leads individuals into the labyrinth of dietary supplements, a landscape teeming with promises of equilibrium and well-being. In this section, we embark on a journey of discovery, separating fact from fiction and guiding you towards evidence-based solutions for hormonal harmony.

Hormonal imbalances are a multifaceted challenge, manifesting in various forms, from irregular menstrual cycles to mood swings that can feel like emotional rollercoasters. The complexity of these issues necessitates a comprehensive approach. Let's begin our exploration by shedding light on some of the supplements that have shown promise in addressing specific hormonal concerns:

Vitex Agnus-Castus: This herbal remedy, also known as Chasteberry, has garnered attention for its potential to regulate menstrual cycles and alleviate symptoms of premenstrual syndrome (PMS). We'll delve into the science behind its effects and how it may offer relief to those navigating the challenges of hormonal fluctuations.

Maca Root: Hailing from the high-altitude Andes, Maca root has gained recognition as an adaptogen with potential benefits for hormonal balance. We'll uncover its unique properties and explore how it can support not only hormonal health but also overall vitality.

Evening Primrose Oil: Often lauded for its gamma-linolenic acid (GLA) content, Evening Primrose Oil has been studied for its role in reducing symptoms of menopause, such as hot flashes and mood swings. We'll provide insights into its mechanisms of action and how it may offer relief during this transformative phase of life.

Adaptogens - Ashwagandha and Rhodiola: In our fast-paced, stress-filled lives, the impact of stress on hormonal balance cannot be overstated. Ashwagandha and Rhodiola, two adaptogenic herbs, take center stage as we explore their ability to mitigate the effects of chronic stress on hormone levels. These adaptogens offer a holistic approach to hormonal well-being.

Omega-3 Fatty Acids: Beyond specific hormonal concerns, inflammation plays a pivotal role in hormonal imbalances. Omega-3 fatty acids, found abundantly in fish oil, hold the potential to quell inflammation and support overall hormonal health. We'll unravel the science behind these essential fatty acids and discuss practical ways to incorporate them into your diet.

Understanding the effectiveness of these supplements requires more than just anecdotal accounts. We'll sift through scientific research and clinical studies to provide you with a comprehensive view of the evidence supporting their use. Each supplement's unique mechanisms of action and potential benefits will be demystified, empowering you to make informed choices on your journey to hormonal balance.

Moreover, we'll emphasize the importance of individualization in supplementation. Your hormonal needs are as unique as you are, and tailoring your supplement regimen to your specific challenges and goals is essential. This section will equip you with the knowledge and tools to make personalized choices that resonate with your body's requirements.

# Understanding Dosages and Quality

Selecting the right supplements is only the first step on your journey to hormonal balance. Equally important is gaining a deep understanding of supplement dosages and ensuring the highest quality standards. In this section, we'll unravel the complexities surrounding supplement dosages and explore the critical importance of quality control.

## Tailoring Dosages to Your Unique Needs

The world of supplements can be overwhelming, with a multitude of options available for every conceivable health concern. To navigate this landscape effectively, it's crucial to tailor your supplement dosages to your individual needs. We're here to demystify this process.

**Personalized Dosages:** There is no one-size-fits-all approach to supplementation. Factors such as age, weight, and specific hormonal concerns play a significant role in determining the right dosage for you. We'll provide you with clear guidelines on how to calculate your ideal dosage based on these variables.

**Hormonal Specifics:** Hormonal imbalances can manifest differently in each individual. Whether you're addressing issues related to estrogen, progesterone, or thyroid hormones, we'll delve into the specific dosages required to target your unique hormonal concerns. Understanding the interplay between different hormones and their impact on your overall well-being is a cornerstone of effective supplementation.

**Health Goals:** Your supplementation needs may evolve as you progress on your journey to hormonal balance. We'll guide you on how to adjust dosages in response to changing health goals, ensuring that you continue to receive the maximum benefits without overloading your system.

**Quality Assurance: Your Health's Best Friend**

Ensuring the quality of the supplements you choose is just as crucial as selecting the right dosages. In this section, we'll underscore the paramount importance of quality control in the world of supplements.

**Reputable Brands:** The supplement market is flooded with a wide range of products, but not all are created equal. We'll provide insights into how to identify reputable brands known for their commitment to quality and safety. This includes researching a company's track record, certifications, and adherence to strict manufacturing standards.

**Reading Labels:** Supplement labels can sometimes appear cryptic, filled with unfamiliar terms and abbreviations. Fear not; we'll guide you through deciphering these labels. You'll learn to recognize key information that indicates the quality of a product, including ingredient lists, dosage specifications, and the presence of third-party certifications.

**Certifications and Testing:** We'll introduce you to the world of third-party testing and certifications. Understanding the significance of certifications like GMP (Good Manufacturing Practices) and NSF (National Sanitation Foundation) will empower you to make informed choices. These certifications ensure that products meet stringent quality and safety standards.

**Product Sourcing:** You'll also gain insights into the importance of where and how supplements are sourced. Discover how factors like ingredient origins, ethical sourcing practices, and sustainability contribute to the overall quality of a supplement.

## Integrating Supplements with Your Diet

Supplements are most potent when seamlessly integrated into your daily diet. In this final section of Chapter 6, we'll delve deeper into the art of harmonizing your dietary choices with your supplement regimen. This integration is where the magic happens, as it allows you to maximize the effectiveness of supplements while savoring delicious and nutritious meals.

***Practical Strategies for Seamlessly Integrating Supplements***

To begin, let's explore practical strategies that will make supplement integration a natural part of your daily routine. The key here is simplicity and consistency. Consider incorporating the following techniques:

**Morning Rituals:** Start your day with a hormone-friendly smoothie or a glass of water infused with supplements like collagen peptides or a high-quality multivitamin. This morning ritual not only jumpstarts your nutrient intake but also sets a positive tone for the day.

**Meal Pairing:** Pair supplements with specific meals. For example, take vitamin D with your breakfast as it enhances calcium absorption. Reserve evening supplements like magnesium for your dinner routine, as they can promote relaxation and restful sleep.

**Snack Time:** Elevate your snacks with nutrient-rich supplements. Nut butter with added omega-3 fatty acids or a handful of almonds paired with vitamin E supplements can turn your snacks into hormonal health boosters.

**Creative Cooking:** Get creative in the kitchen by incorporating supplements into your cooking. Stir collagen powder into your soups and stews for added protein and skin support. Experiment with turmeric supplements in curries for their anti-inflammatory properties.

**Supplement-Focused Recipes:** Explore our collection of supplement-focused recipes tailored to your hormonal balance goals. From hormone-balancing smoothies bursting with antioxidants to nutrient-dense salads topped with fertility-supporting supplements, these recipes are designed to make supplement intake delicious and enjoyable.

# CHAPTER 7

# BEYOND DIET: LIFESTYLE CHANGES FOR HORMONAL HEALTH

## Exercise and Its Impact on Hormones

Exercise is a powerful tool that can significantly influence hormonal balance in women. While the benefits of regular physical activity extend far beyond weight management, it's essential to understand the intricate relationship between exercise and hormones.

### The Hormonal Response to Exercise

When you engage in physical activity, your body releases a cascade of hormones, each playing a specific role. For instance, endorphins, often referred to as "feel-good hormones," are released during exercise, contributing to a sense of well-being and reducing stress. Additionally, exercise can help regulate insulin levels, which is crucial for blood sugar control.

### Hormonal Balance Through Different Types of Exercise

Not all exercise is created equal when it comes to hormonal health. Different forms of exercise can have varying impacts on hormones. For example, aerobic exercises like running or cycling can enhance cardiovascular health and boost endorphin production. Strength training, on the other hand, can promote muscle growth and improve metabolism.

## Exercise and Hormonal Conditions

Exercise can be especially beneficial for women dealing with hormonal conditions like Polycystic Ovary Syndrome (PCOS) and menopause. In PCOS, regular exercise can help improve insulin sensitivity and regulate menstrual cycles. For menopausal women, exercise can mitigate some of the symptoms such as hot flashes and mood swings.

## The Importance of Balance

While exercise is a potent tool for hormonal health, it's essential to strike a balance. Overtraining or excessive exercise without proper recovery can lead to hormonal imbalances. Understanding your body's signals and adopting a sustainable exercise routine is key.

## Stress Management Techniques

Stress is an unavoidable part of modern life, but its chronic presence can wreak havoc on hormonal balance. Understanding how stress affects hormones and learning effective stress management techniques is crucial for overall well-being.

## The Stress-Hormone Connection

Stress triggers the release of cortisol, often referred to as the "stress hormone." While cortisol is essential for the body's fight-or-flight response, chronic stress can lead to an overproduction of cortisol, disrupting hormonal balance. This can result in symptoms such as anxiety, sleep disturbances, and weight gain.

## Mind-Body Techniques for Stress Reduction

Numerous mind-body techniques have been proven to reduce stress and rebalance hormones. These include practices like mindfulness meditation, deep breathing exercises, and yoga. These practices promote relaxation, lower cortisol levels, and improve overall hormonal health.

## Lifestyle Modifications

Managing stress isn't limited to meditation and yoga; lifestyle choices also play a significant role. Adequate social support, time management, and setting boundaries are essential for stress reduction. Moreover, engaging in hobbies and activities you enjoy can have a positive impact on your mood and stress levels.

## The Role of Nutrition

Dietary choices can either exacerbate or alleviate stress. Consuming a balanced diet rich in nutrients can support the body's stress response. Certain foods, like those high in omega-3 fatty acids and antioxidants, can help reduce inflammation and improve mood.

# The Importance of Sleep

Sleep is often underestimated when considering hormonal health, yet it plays a pivotal role in regulating hormones. Understanding the significance of sleep and adopting healthy sleep habits is essential for hormonal balance.

## The Sleep-Hormone Connection

During sleep, the body undergoes crucial processes for hormonal regulation and overall well-being. Growth hormone, which is vital for tissue repair and metabolism, is primarily released during deep sleep stages. Additionally, sleep influences the balance of hormones like cortisol, insulin, and leptin, which affect appetite and stress response.

## The Impact of Sleep Deprivation

Chronic sleep deprivation disrupts the delicate balance of hormones. It can lead to increased cortisol levels, insulin resistance, and changes in appetite-regulating hormones, ultimately contributing to weight gain and hormonal imbalances. Sleep deficiency is also linked to mood disorders and cognitive impairment.

## Establishing Healthy Sleep Patterns

Creating healthy sleep patterns is essential for hormonal health. This includes maintaining a consistent sleep schedule, creating a conducive sleep environment, and practicing relaxation techniques before bedtime. Limiting exposure to screens and caffeine in the evening can also improve sleep quality.

## Sleep and Hormonal Conditions

Women dealing with hormonal conditions like menopause or irregular menstrual cycles may find that improving sleep quality can alleviate some of their symptoms. Sleep is a natural regulator of hormonal fluctuations, and optimizing sleep can contribute to greater hormonal balance.

# CHAPTER 8

## SPECIAL CONSIDERATIONS

## Managing PCOS and Endometriosis Through Diet

Polycystic Ovary Syndrome (PCOS) and endometriosis are two common yet challenging conditions that many women face. While diet alone may not be a cure, it can play a significant role in managing symptoms and improving overall quality of life.

### Understanding PCOS and Endometriosis:

PCOS is characterized by hormonal imbalances, insulin resistance, and the presence of cysts on the ovaries. Endometriosis, on the other hand, involves the growth of tissue similar to the lining of the uterus outside the uterus, causing pain and fertility issues. Both conditions can lead to chronic pain, irregular menstrual cycles, and fertility challenges.

### The Role of Diet:

Diet can influence these conditions in several ways. For PCOS, managing insulin levels through a balanced diet can be key. This means choosing complex carbohydrates over refined sugars, incorporating lean proteins, and opting for healthy fats. For endometriosis, an anti-inflammatory diet rich in fruits, vegetables, whole grains, and omega-3 fatty acids may help reduce inflammation and pain.

**Balancing Hormones:**

Certain foods can have a positive impact on hormonal balance. Fiber-rich foods like broccoli, flaxseeds, and lentils can help regulate estrogen levels, which is crucial in managing both PCOS and endometriosis. Additionally, antioxidants from colorful fruits and vegetables can combat oxidative stress often seen in these conditions.

**Avoiding Triggers:**

Some foods may exacerbate symptoms. For PCOS, it's essential to limit processed foods and excess sugar, as they can worsen insulin resistance. For endometriosis, foods that can promote inflammation, such as red meat and dairy, may need to be minimized.

**Herbal Supplements:**

Certain herbs and supplements like cinnamon, inosltol, and turmeric have shown promise in managing PCOS symptoms. Similarly, natural anti-inflammatories like curcumin and quercetin may provide relief for those with endometriosis.

**Lifestyle Factors:** Beyond diet, maintaining a healthy weight through regular exercise is crucial for both conditions. Weight management can help regulate hormones and reduce the severity of symptoms.

# Diet During Menopause and Perimenopause

Menopause is a natural part of a woman's life, marking the end of reproductive years. Perimenopause is the transitional period leading up to menopause and can bring about a range of physical and emotional changes. Diet plays a vital role in supporting women through this transition.

## Hormonal Changes:

During perimenopause and menopause, there is a significant shift in hormone levels, particularly estrogen. This hormonal fluctuation can lead to hot flashes, mood swings, weight gain, and bone density loss.

## Bone Health:

Maintaining bone health is a primary concern during this stage. A diet rich in calcium and vitamin D is essential to support bone density. Foods like dairy, leafy greens, and fortified cereals can help. Additionally, resistance training can strengthen bones.

## Heart Health:

With hormonal changes comes an increased risk of heart disease. A heart-healthy diet involves reducing saturated fats and incorporating more monounsaturated fats found in nuts and olive oil. Omega-3 fatty acids from fatty fish like salmon can also protect the heart.

**Weight Management:**

Metabolism tends to slow down during menopause, making weight management challenging. A balanced diet that controls portion sizes and includes lean proteins, whole grains, and plenty of vegetables can help maintain a healthy weight.

**Managing Hot Flashes:**

Certain foods, like caffeine and spicy foods, can trigger hot flashes. Limiting these triggers and staying hydrated can help minimize discomfort.

**Mood and Brain Health:**

Omega-3 fatty acids, found in fatty fish and flaxseeds, may support mood and cognitive function during menopause. B-vitamins from whole grains and leafy greens are also important for brain health.

## Addressing Thyroid Imbalances with Nutrition

The thyroid is a small gland with a mighty influence on the body's metabolism and overall health. Thyroid imbalances, such as hypothyroidism (underactive thyroid) and hyperthyroidism (overactive thyroid), can be managed and supported through dietary choices.

**Understanding Thyroid Imbalances:**

Hypothyroidism can lead to fatigue, weight gain, and depression, while hyperthyroidism can cause weight loss, anxiety, and heart palpitations. Diet can help mitigate these symptoms.

**Iodine and Selenium:**

Iodine is a crucial component of thyroid hormones. Incorporating iodized salt and iodine-rich foods like seafood is important for thyroid health. Selenium, found in nuts and seeds, helps regulate thyroid function and can reduce inflammation.

**Goitrogens:**

Goitrogens are compounds found in certain foods like broccoli, cauliflower, and kale that can interfere with thyroid function when consumed in excess. Cooking these foods can reduce their goitrogenic properties.

**Limiting Processed Foods:**

Processed foods often contain unhealthy fats, excessive salt, and additives that can disrupt thyroid function. Opting for whole, unprocessed foods is beneficial.

**Balancing Nutrients:** Ensuring an adequate intake of vitamins and minerals like vitamin D, B-vitamins, and zinc is essential for thyroid health. These nutrients can be obtained from a varied and balanced diet.

**Food Sensitivities:**

Some individuals with thyroid imbalances may have sensitivities to gluten or dairy. Identifying and avoiding these trigger foods can help alleviate symptoms.

# CONCLUSION

As we conclude this exploration of the Hormonal Balance Diet for Women, I invite you to reflect on the power of food in shaping not only our physical health but also our emotional well-being and vitality. Throughout this journey, we've delved into the intricate world of women's health, dissecting the role of hormones and how they influence our lives in profound ways.

From understanding the hormonal symphony that orchestrates our bodies to embracing a diet that nourishes our unique needs, we've traveled a path paved with knowledge and practicality. We've seen how diet can be a beacon of hope for those grappling with conditions like PCOS and endometriosis, offering strategies to manage symptoms and regain control.

In the throes of perimenopause and menopause, we've explored how diet can ease the transition, supporting bone health, heart health, and emotional balance. We've uncovered the secrets to thriving during these transformative phases of life.

And in the realm of thyroid imbalances, we've witnessed the influence of nutrients like iodine and selenium, as well as the importance of mindful food choices in nurturing thyroid health.

But this journey is not confined to the pages of this book; it's a lifelong expedition. The Hormonal Balance Diet is more than a set of guidelines; it's an invitation to take charge of your health, to savor the flavors of life while honoring the needs of your body.

As you embark on this path, remember that your journey is unique. Your body is a tapestry of experiences, and what serves as nourishment for one may not be the same for another. Embrace the flexibility to tailor this diet to your individual needs, consult with healthcare professionals, and listen to the wisdom of your body.

Through the stories, insights, and practical advice shared in these pages, you hold the keys to a healthier, more harmonious life. The Hormonal Balance Diet for Women is more than a diet; it's an empowering journey toward holistic well-being, where you are the author of your health story.

May this knowledge be your companion as you navigate the labyrinth of women's health, may it inspire you to make choices that honor your body, and may it empower you to lead a life of vitality and balance.

With every meal, every bite, and every mindful choice, you have the power to transform not just your hormones, but your life. Embrace this journey, for it is a celebration of your health, your strength, and your radiant spirit.

Here's to the Hormonal Balance Diet for Women—a journey to a healthier, happier you.